HOW TO
ATTRACT THE
RIGHT PEOPLE
IN 90 SECONDS

Simple & easy tricks to become more attractive

Mr. Dheeraj D. Rathod

PREFACE

My dear friends,

I am extremely elated to present to you the book "How to attract the right people in 90 Seconds ". This book speaks through the stories and situational flashes of images. It's Small chapters and highly precise content makes it more interesting, engaging and understandable to a reader.

I am thankful to the Glucotech Team for the encouragement and support that they have extended and I am also thankful to my friends for their efforts to make this book as good as it can be. We have jointly made every possible effort to eliminate all the errors in this book.

However if you come across any, please do let us know, because that will surely help us to improve this work further to make it more enjoyable. I would also extend my gratitude towards Ishwari Dawkhar for placing all the commas and the full stops in their appropriate places and making the content of the book grammatically correct. I would also like to thank Sanjana Tickoo for lending her sweet voice to the narration of this book for the audience of my

audible book.   I would like to thank Abhishek Sandbhor for using the best of his skills for the formatting.
I am also thankful to my family members for their encouragement and patience.

Mr. Dheeraj Dashrath Rathod

CONTENTS

INTRODUCTION

I believe this book will explain all the possible secrets of making a good impression, pro trips for pleasantly and impactfully conversing with everyone. This will help in establishing instant rapport, to build good relations and will entitle you as the most charismatic person in the room.

This book is written by observing highly influential personalities from different walks of life. It is a secret pro tip to reveal the worst and the best of you smartly and influence people around you.

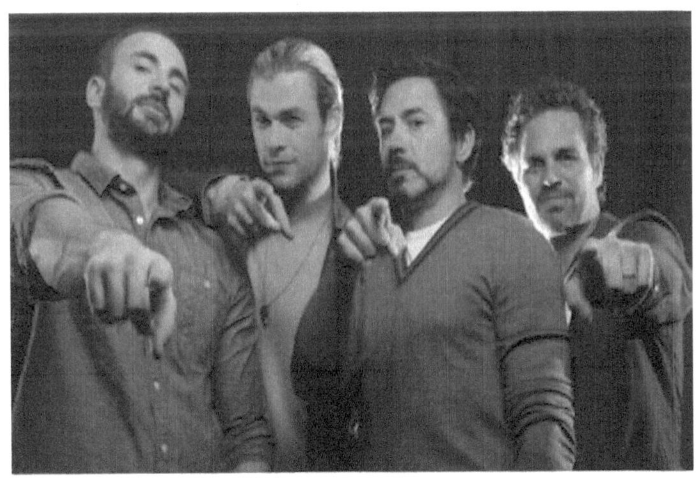

All person to person interactions and business relationships are based on body language, rapport building and communication skills. The key to establish quick rapport is to synchronize conversational behaviour and make the first impression.

There are many such secret tricks that will make your personality attractive. It is often said, 'Don't judge a book by its cover', but in today's world, a positively influential personality makes its way through people's attention. No matter what inner qualities the person possesses other than a dashing personality, he is already marked up in the rank of potentially good candidates in the very first impression.

This is also known as an inner positive 'aura', which you will learn to harness through this book. Being certain that someone likes you or finds you attractive already wins you half the battle!

Three simple secrets and you are half done:

- ➤ Psychological Secret: Which Psychological tricks make a person more attractive?
- ➤ **Body Language Secret:** What body language basics do attractive personalities frequently use?

- **Communication Secret:** How to have a simple yet effective communication session to create instant trust as well as a strong rapport.

Psychological Secret

1-Trust Mirror

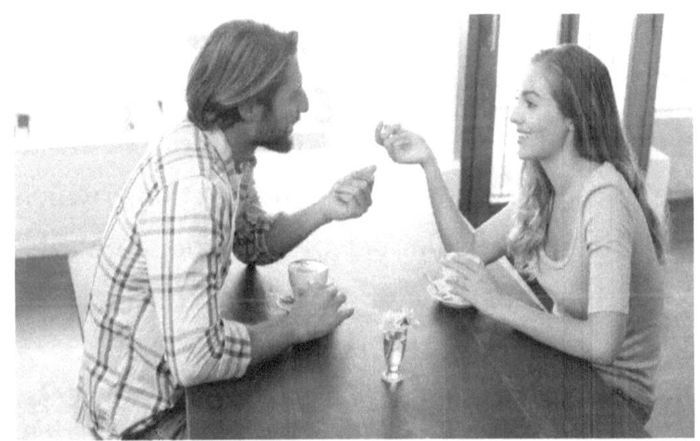

Trust is the foundation of an unfailing and dependable business as well as a personal relationship. If you want to earn people's trust more quickly, then a trust mirror can be a very effective method of doing so.

When you're striking a conversation with people, try mirroring their body language. Don't do this in an incredibly obvious way; otherwise it'll probably put them off more than anything else.

However, subtly mirroring people's body language subconsciously makes them think you're in sync, which works very well for building mutual trust.

Several studies show that we are more likely to help those who dress like us. Actions which depict that a particular person is on the same page boosts the trust factor and can do marvels, especially in business relationships. This is a master trick to get people to trust you with all sorts of investments like time, money and even emotions.

2- Warm Hands

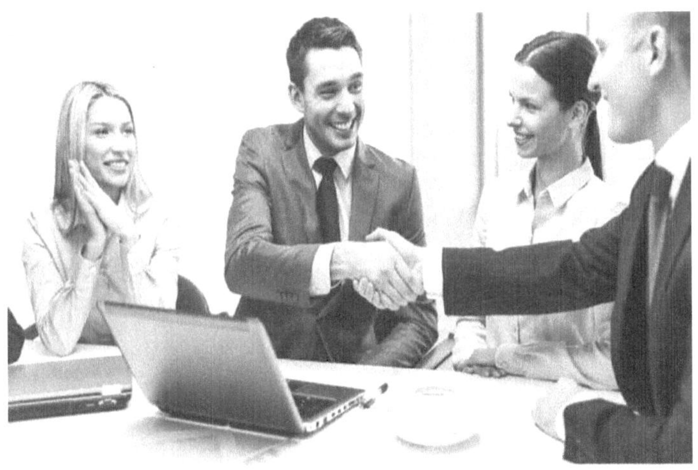

When you shake hands for the first time, try and make sure you have warm hands. Warms hands means a warm and welcoming approach to an introduction.

This makes you far more impressive and attractive to the other person, no matter who they are. Cold hands symbolize a cold and poor introduction.

This brings up the point of not vigorously rubbing your cold hands in front of the other person to make them warm as it would make the person in front of you uncomfortable. Instead, take a minute aside to warm up your hands before going forward for a welcoming hand shake.

Do not make anything regarding your body language too obvious as it would put off your impression. Remember, 'First impression is the only impression' when it comes to personality and outgoingness.

3- Eye Contact

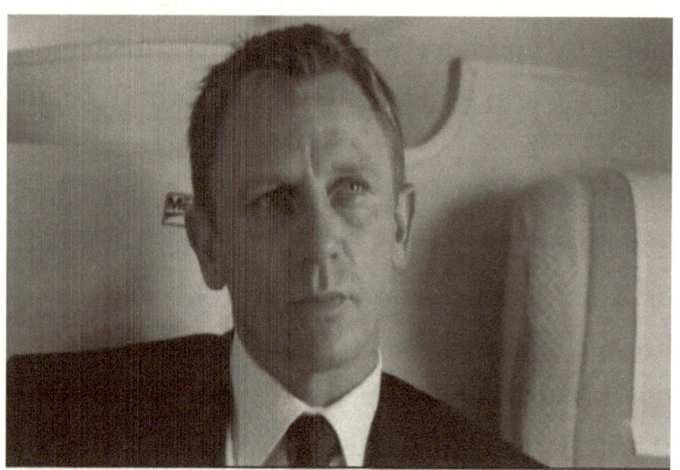

It has been aptly said that eyes are the window to the soul. Of course we all are aware about this fact but how many of us truly understand its importance?

We rarely work towards establishing eye contact in our daily conversations. Having a steady eye contact signifies a positive attitude, depicts purity as well as clarity of thought. Additionally it also shows that you are fearless and are giving importance to the person with whom you are having a legitimate conversation.

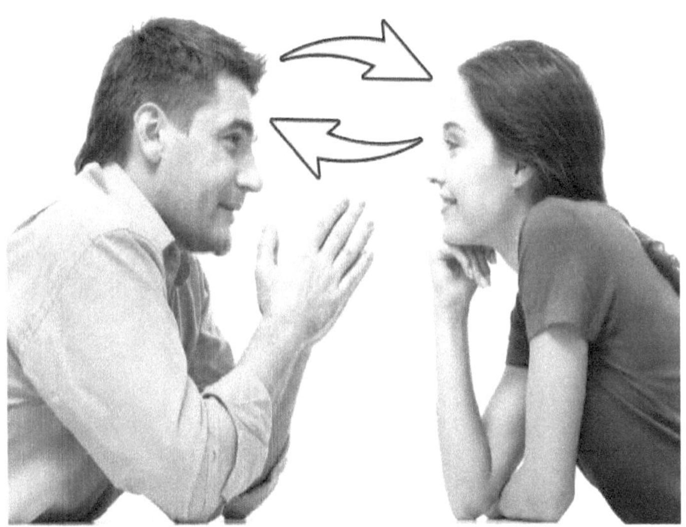

Many people find it hard to maintain eye contact. In fact, most people find it very uncomfortable to maintain eye contact, not necessarily while listening, but also while speaking. However, you can start practicing eye contact by being genuinely alert and responsive of the other person's words.

Another very important conversation etiquette is to avoid checking your mobile phone for constant message notifications or general screen scrolling. This depicts sheer disinterest for the speaker who is trying to pitch a conversation.

Hence, avoid answering messages unless they are meant to be addressed urgently. This is how you can be a good listener. A good and attentive listener is always appreciated and puts up a fantastic first impression.

4- A good sense of humor

A good sense of humour is generally associated with intelligence and honesty. That's why humorous people are always the favorite ones in the room.

A humorous person can light up the room with a heartfelt laughter and can distress any heated up situation very easily. Humour extensively portrays positivity and liveliness and thus is an eminent trait in attractive and positive influencer personalities.

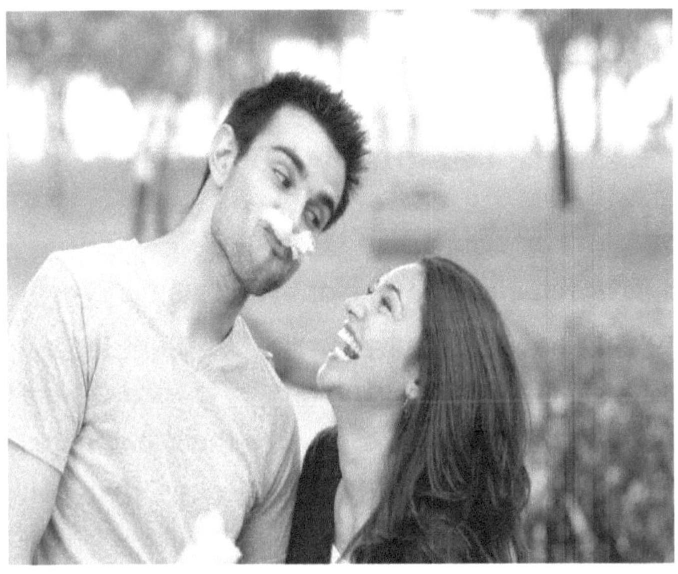

Being humorous portrays a healthy state of mind! At the same time, it should also be noted that forced humour is the most unwelcoming gesture. If you feel that your humour fails to hit the tickle bones of people you converse with, do not overdo your jokes or funny comments as it can put off the mood of a light hearted conversation.

Being funny is definitely a key to attract people, but forced humour can result in ignorance from people around you. Every individual is the best in his or her own way and embracing it is the most intelligent move.

5- Calling Person by their Real Name

Always remember a person's first name. It will prove to be the sweetest gesture for any person and will stay with them always.

When you address a person with their first name, it gives him or her a pleasant feeling that you remember how they made you feel and that always works as an advantage to create a great bond.

Remembering names, at the same time, can be as tough as finding a needle in a heap of dry hay for some people. That is why do not fumble when you do not remember a person's name in the second meeting, just talk normally and casually and then ask for his or her card or phone number. Keeping the conversation light hearted without getting nervous can always be a great escape. While asking for the person' s contact number, be polite and ask , "How do you spell your name?" rather than asking ," What is your name?". This trick works almost every time only if you maintain the vibe of the conversation.

6- Compliment People on what they have earned

Let's be honest! We all crave for compliments. We all tend to like a person who keeps complimenting us often over a person who compliments very occasionally.

In this hustle of life, each individual is striving hard to achieve great milestones with dedication and hardwork. This stands true for all aspects including career. Therefore take time to appreciate people and their achievements. This gives people a positive notion about you and they tend to have a positive approach towards you immediately.

Appreciating and complimenting people doesn't take much. It may be anything, like an impressive physique, their fashionable clothing sense, a beautiful smile, a haircut that makes them look groomed. You can also congratulate people on their achievement, on a personal as well as professional front.

Giving compliments makes people feel good and confident about themselves. Let's see how you can make a difference in a person's life by a simple compliment.

- A positive comment encourages a gloomy person to be an enthusiastic one. A compliment can make a person's day and might be the best thing they hear about themselves while coping up with a tough day. Paying a compliment also uplifts our mood as the more positively we talk to others, the more positive our approach towards the day bends to be. Hence learn to pay a compliment to make someone and yourself feel great.

- It is a basic tendency of human creatures to be suckers for flattery.

- A very important thing to be noted is that only genuine compliments make it to people's hearts. Be genuine ! For example, if you do not like a person's choice of shirt , don't go out of the way and praise them for that. People can quickly identify buttery compliments. Buttery compliments portray the person as untruthful which by default results in a negative impression. We personally do not fall for false compliments hence we should respect the same for other individuals around us as well. False compliments if paid to your seniors may land into trouble as you would be soon coined as the 'boss's pet' by your work colleagues and honestly, no one looks forward to that.

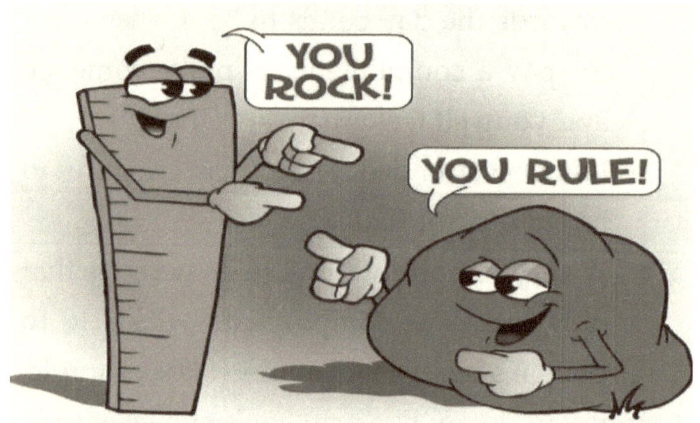

7- Become a Great Storyteller

Storytelling is the ability to captivate a person or a group of people with an engaging narrative that charms them. Effective storytelling will make the listeners feel like they are a part of the story.

People remember stories far beyond facts and figures. Storytelling is one of the most important skills you should learn in your life. This is the reason why movies tend to influence so many people as movies are an visually appealing interpretation of stories.

Therefore it makes sense that stories can bring together people of different tastes and interests. Stories are a gateway to a person's inner creativity and a reflection of his soul.

The best way to know a person is to know him through the stories he narrates and the way he narrates them. You can leave a person bewitched and spell bound by your story by maintaining a pleasant eye contact.

The Art Of Story Telling

8- To share your deepest secrets

The most important law of instant attraction is to tell people your deepest secrets by looking in their eyes. Bollywood, in its songs has the best description on this law; e.g. Naina thug lenge, thug lenge naina,

English songs also have similar instances. Taylor Swift says "Your beautiful eyes, stare right into my eyes. And sometimes I think of you late at night, I don't know why."

The very famous Urdu Shayar Mirza Ghalib said "Hum to Fana Ho Gaye Unki Aankhen Dekhkar Galib, Na Jane wo Aaina Kaise Dekhate Honge."

This translates as "I got lost in the bewitched eyes, I wonder how the eyes reflect my truth"

If the secrets you share come from your within, maintaining eye contact and making the listener believe them is not a tough job.

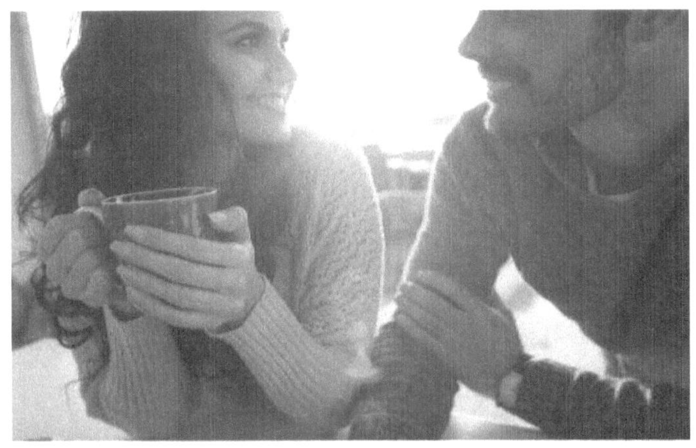

9- Don't Be Afraid To Break the Rules

Let's consider a common scenario. If a Polo shirt and cotton pants are your uniform, many of you tend to wear it anywhere and everywhere. But being occasional and clothing friendly is the smartness of attractive people.

You should try things out of your comfort zone. This is one of the laws which is ritually followed by the most attractive people in the world.

You can browse your favorite personality from any walk of life. It is a fact that only rule breakers can be trendsetters and trendsetters are the ones who influence people positively.

Rules are meant to be broken sometimes, especially when you feel that they are overpowering your way of existence. Do not hesitate in breaking rules. Break rules only when you are absolutely certain about yourself. The first step of self-exploration is breaking rules and creating positive disruptions in the chain of events.

10- Smile with eye contact is a perfect law of attraction

The person who makes eye contact with us while smiling is always unforgettable. Such a moment gets registered as good feelings in our mind. If we recall these moments, we will naturally see ourselves smiling in the mirror. Such moments become a topic for our sweet dreams. Hey! There you go ! I caught you, didn't I ? Keep blushing and do not be shy, it is normal and beautiful.

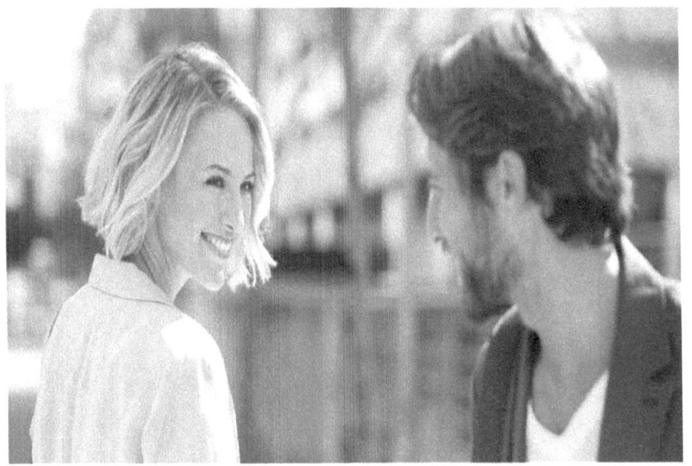

11- Positive appearance

It is a modern trend that appearances are trusted upon more by today's human beings than the sincerity of a person's character. Attractiveness and honest appearance can easily be misleading. Here is an example to prove the above point. Whenever you interact during a business meeting, you tend to influence people and make a long-lasting impression on them with the way you carry yourself and break the ice with your conversation etiquettes.

This means that your work, achievements and promotions are not significant when you make a first impression. You do not hang your promotion letter or trophies around your neck and roam around.

So, to be a head turner at such events, it is very important to carry yourself well. You should groom yourself in such a way that it will emit the confidence you behold within.

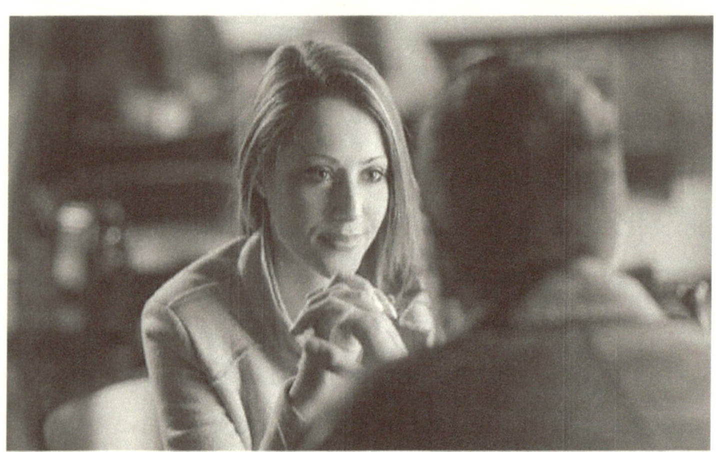

12- Social value is extremely powerful and makes you more attractive

A man surrounded by crowds seems very attractive to women. In the same way, a majority of men do not prefer ladies who are airheaded but fall for women who are interactive and cheerfully light up the room with their energy and smile.

Generally speaking, the social value of the opposite gender matters to most of us. Social value means how accepting one is to society and how acceptance is reverted back by society towards him. This is definitely not written to target introverted or socially inept individuals as introversion in their behaviour is their personal choice.

Moreover, even if you are the life of a party, no one gives you a right to question anybody's outlook towards life and otherwise. This is written to address people who want to break through their comfort zone and explore themselves thoroughly.

Here's an example. In a research carried out in 2010, a group of researchers from Duke University asked a group of heterosexual volunteers to rate the attractiveness of men and women who were photographed by themselves. The researchers then showed a second group of volunteers pictures of the same men and women, but this time paired with a person of the opposite sex whom the volunteers told were their ex-partners'. Their findings come forth as; the men and women who were photographed next to a "hot" ex's were almost always rated as more attractive by the volunteers from the second group, even if they weren't rated as highly by volunteers from the first group. You can read more about this effect here.

13- Surrounded by the opposite Gender

The best indicator of a man worth a woman spending her time with is if other women are already spending their time with him.

Being popular with the ladies can be actually a good thing! If women see other females spending time with you, it seems like you are worthy of their time. This will definitely attract more females.

The same theory applies for females as well. If men see a woman hanging out with a couple of men, they are instantly attracted towards her. This simple logic seems very pretentious but stands very true.

14- Leadership skills are attractive in your social life.

Leaders and quality of leadership have been glorified in human history since ages. It is not a myth but it is the truth that leaders carry some charm that makes them attractive.

Men who make great leaders enchant women easily. It is a truth we all have to accept at some time or the other in our career phase that the corporate world is majorly male-dominated.

Dynamic women are breaking this stereotype in all walks of life and it is a psychological truth that some men are crippled with an inferiority complex when it comes to strong, influential women leading them. But, to a pleasant contrary, a true gentleman acknowledges the leadership and competition from everyone and supports healthy competition.

This quality of men is highly appreciated by strong-headed women. Strong headed women do not approach men who they feel are insecure of women with their aura and achievements. Instead, men who openly stand by women with power eventually make it to their hearts as well (not necessarily always, therefore let's accept this, women already have a civilization of men trying their luck on them.)

Leadership is not only possessing the ability to lead but also bonding and respecting your team well to strive together towards great ambitions and goals. Leadership depends on the sheer understanding ability of an individual and both, men and women make the best of leaders if they possess the qualities and spirit for it. At the end of the day, the one who leads, is the one who binds the team together.

Leadership qualities make an individual positively influential and trustworthy, not only in terms of professional accomplishments but also in terms of personal accomplishments.

15- Being Passionate and Versatile

Have you ever heard someone speak passionately about something and ended up being totally unaware of what was going on around you, and became completely absorbed by their presence?

Passionate individuals drive people crazy, in a good way. Passionate people are one of the best people to be around. People who are passionate understand the true meaning of life and believe in living for every fleeting moment. These individuals make the best of opportunities given in their basket of luck.

A stagnant water pond is a breeding ground for insects and foul smell and fails to serve the purpose of liveliness, serenity and purity. Non Versalite people are like stagnant ponds as they attract only people with the same amount of non-versatility and disinterest towards life. Non versatile people avoid experimenting and exploring themselves and thus lack an open minded approach towards life and otherwise. Such people are usually difficult to be around and work with, hence, they end up being lonely.

16- Look for someone 'in your league'

Men and women naturally get attracted to people who are as attractive as they are. The basic psychology behind this is that people match with wavelengths. The popular saying-"Your vibe attracts your tribe" is very true in this sense.

So, if you find someone who shares the same wavelength and views as you, hold on to them. Learn things from them and try to match with them which will make you more attractive.

17- Husky Voice prevails always!

Words are the most important medium of expression of our thoughts, ideas and emotions. The ability of verbal expression makes us as humans, very privileged over other creations of God.

However, the ability to deliver a pleasant speech is an art indeed. If you ask any woman who is more attractive- David Beckham or John Hamm (based on their voices alone), there is a greater chance that she'll pick John.

But why is it that women in general seem to find men with deeper, huskier voices more attractive? Well, according to few researchers from University College London, it's because women perceive a deeper voice as a sign of a larger and stronger physicality; something that women are evolutionarily geared to find attractive.

Similarly, men get attracted to the sweet and pleasant voices of women and thus get influenced in a positive way. It's not possible to change your vocal chords to make you sound huskier or shriller, so rely more on the quality of speech!

18- Finger length

In recent years scientists have discovered that there is an intriguing link between finger length and the levels of testosterone that a man was exposed to while still in the womb. A longer ring finger indicates increased testosterone.

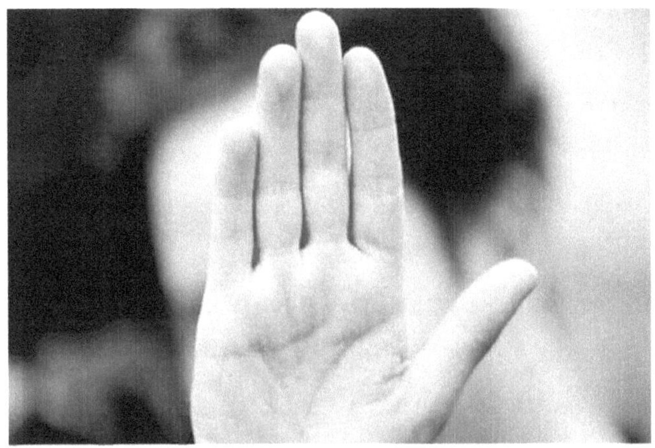

19- We look for qualities that our parents possess opposite Gender

Since ages it has been observed that children find attachment with the parents of their opposite sex. E.g. a son will always feel close to his mother whereas a daughter tends to be the father's favourite. Some research also suggests that we are prone to find people who look like our opposite sex parent attractive.

According to research from St Andrews, we are attracted to the features that our parents had when we were born, possibly because we see them as our first caregiver, and associate positive feelings with their features.

Also, in a follow up study, a sample of 697 men and women showed people were more likely to have romantic partners who had the same eye and hair color as their opposite-sex parents.

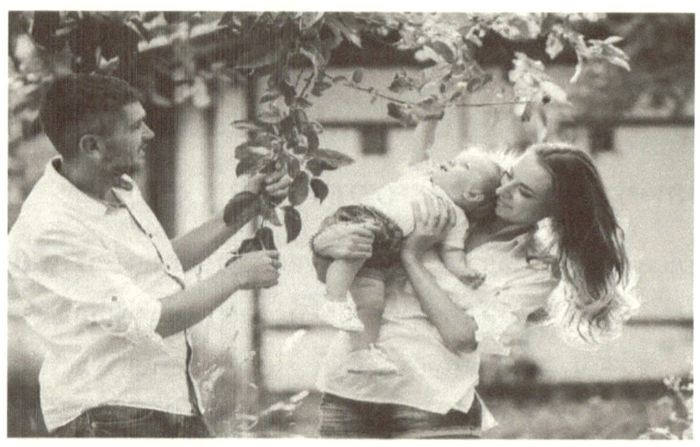

20- Being Mysterious and Unpredictable

It is often believed that most love marriages or love affairs do not tend to last for a 'forever' because the partners involved in the relationship end up getting bored of each other's company.

It is very often said that our better half should know us in and out to be in a healthy relationship, but this is partially true. You should always keep a part of yourself open for exploration rather than putting it all out at once.

Mysteries excite people and hence keep them intact with you for a long time. This holds true for not only romantic relationships, but also for all types of relationships we build in our lives.

Relationship building is an art , if done right, it can make your life more interesting and full of great experiences with all types of people.

Here are a few easy ways to be unpredictable with people you've just met. It's as simple as this:

- Don't do what other people do. Remember, never go where the crowd goes and never join a line which others join, instead , find your own path and make your own line. The destination may be the same, but at the end, it's the journey to that destination that counts. It's the journey that makes us different from others. It's the journey that makes reaching the destination worth it. Hence, explore your path in your own way.

- Don't tell people what you're going to do. First step to pursue unpredictability is not letting out your ideas or future plans. This way your ideas and thoughts are less prone to get copied and implemented by another individual before you. And this always tends to grab the other person's interest and attention in your talks. In this world of social media where everyone is engrossed in being pretentious, maintaining your mystery will certainly make you stand out. Letting others discover and unveil your qualities eventually proves that you're genuinely an interesting person to be around with.

- Keep escalating things, move fast, and make headway contrasting qualities that stimulate curiosity. Let's agree to not disagree with this fact, we all love surprises and look forward to them, especially the ones which are non-occasional as they make us feel special, loved and most importantly wanted. Attractive and positively influential people tend to keep a close eye on your likes and dislikes and make an effort to give you non occasional as well as occasional surprises. They are by far the best surprises you would receive from anyone. Reciprocating love, attention and concern in any relationship can help an individual bond with his/her partner more beautifully. It will also make the relationship strong enough to withstand all odds of life.

***

Body Language

1- Posture

Body language provides an amazing amount of information of what others are thinking about you. It is aptly said that a person having a positive and upright body language gives out positive energy which can make others around you adapt or correct their body language.

Body language makes you a recipient of a lot of positive and uplighting comments from your work colleagues. It is a master key to influence people positively and attract and captivate their attention towards you in a good way.

Research has shown that we automatically assign good-looking individuals favorable traits such as talent, kindness, honesty, friendliness, intelligence and so on. This is called the Halo effect. Oh and we do this without being aware that physical attractiveness plays a role in this process.

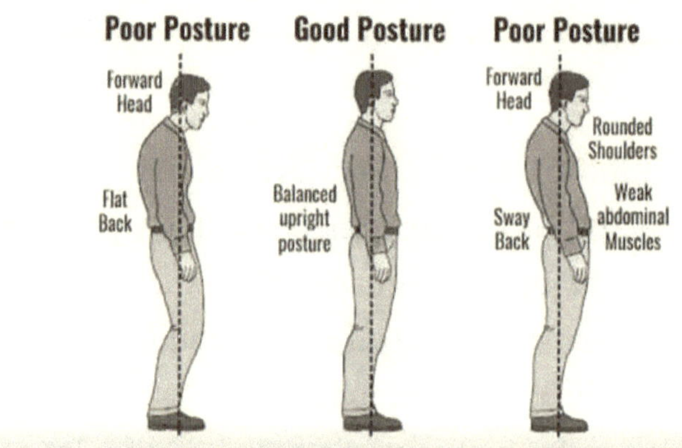

2- Open Body Language

Open body language is positioning yourself in a way that makes you look more approachable and friendly as opposed to a closed body language. Closed body language is positioning you in a way that drives people away from you.

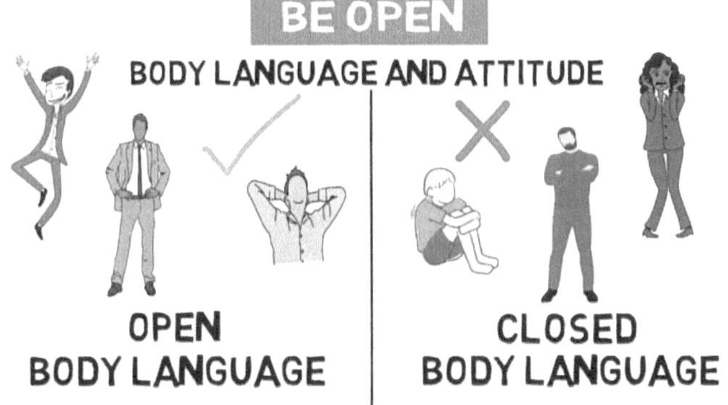

3- Upright positioned Torso

For an upright positioned torso, your shoulder should be rolled back and upright, it makes the chest look bigger and tight.

A slouchy body language fails to put up a good long-lasting impression on others. No matter how diligently you deliver a speech or presentation in front of your audience, bad torso posture fails to make the expected impact which is always heartbreaking and sometimes even embarrassing.

4- Chin and Head

A proper posture of head and chin shows confidence. Did you ever observe that to get a perfect click, the cameraman asks you to pull your chin up and hold your head straight?

It is a secret that is ritually followed by men and women who find it attractive in other people. Once you hold your head straight, you naturally succeed in maintaining comfortable eye contact with the person in front of you. This gives a welcoming impression about you to the other person.

The golden rule of public speaking is to hold your head and chin straight and to maintain eye contact with the audience to have them in sync with your speech.

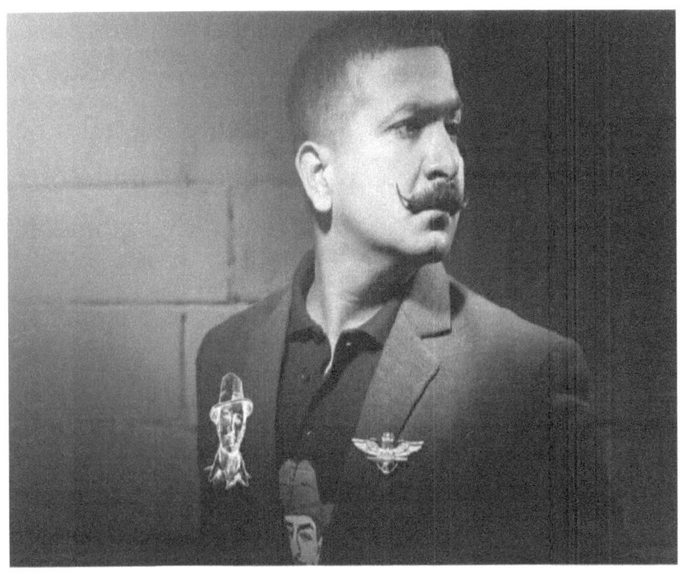

5- Forward looking Eyes

Maintaining your eye level might be one of the trickiest ways to show confidence in body language. When you're walking anywhere by yourself, it often feels natural to lower your head slightly and watch your step, but this posture communicates to others that you don't want to engage in conversation or interact.

It also communicates 'inferiority complex, anxiety, stress, fear and low confidence.' And if you're not careful, you might get into the habit of doing it all the time. Keep your chin up and your eyes forward, even when you're walking alone on the street.

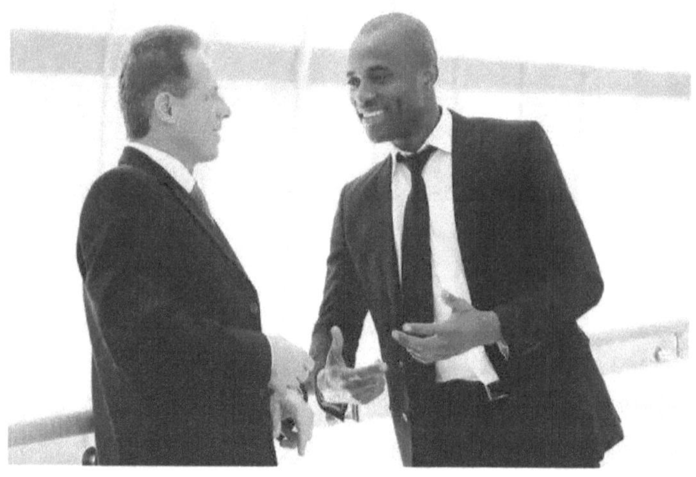

Just look at them for a couple of seconds in a mature way.

What have you understood? Write in your own word

here____

6- Flash a Generous Smile

Who wants a company of dull faces surrounding them throughout the day? Of course, none of us, not at all! But, why?

Dull faced people don't ignite warmth and comfort. A person with a generous smile will impress anyone right away. Many attractive people are experts in the 'beam' smile. What it means is that letting your cheek muscles flex wide apart resulting in a broad smile.

This happens not because the smiling people don't have nothing to worry about but just because they know the value of it. To be an attractive ambassador of a smile to all those who you meet, see, and pass by you. In such a case chances of getting a return smile and a blessing is very high.

Smiles and laughter are contagious. In this world where everyone have their eye sights locked on a screen of a smart phone which ironically is making us dumb day by day, no one really cares to exchange this token of friendliness.

It is ironic how we end up using more 'emojis' in our chat window than our real lives. We exchange those cute smiley emojis to any other person on our chat list but are hesitant to do the same in real life. The sad truth is that we are 'textually' very approachable but struggle to be 'socially' approachable.

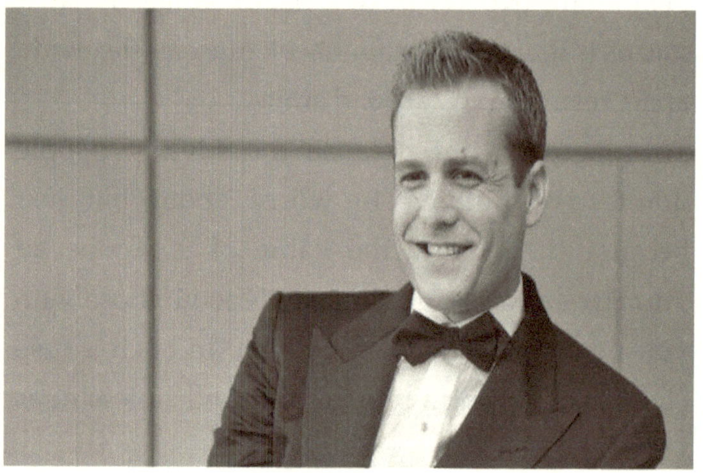

7- Firm handshake

A firm and solid handshake is a symbol of an intelligent, smart, and attractive individual. It is worse than reaching out to one's hand during introduction or welcome and you find a limp noodle. A firm handshake speaks volumes about your personality, upbringing, and company of people you are surrounded by.

Instead, grab the other person's hand firmly and confidently. If shaking hands with someone you've already met, you might even consider the two-hand grab: placing your free hand on the other person's elbow adds warmth and enthusiasm to the handshake.

Just don't get carried away. A handshake is not a contest. Don't try to crush the other person's hand and don't hold on too long.

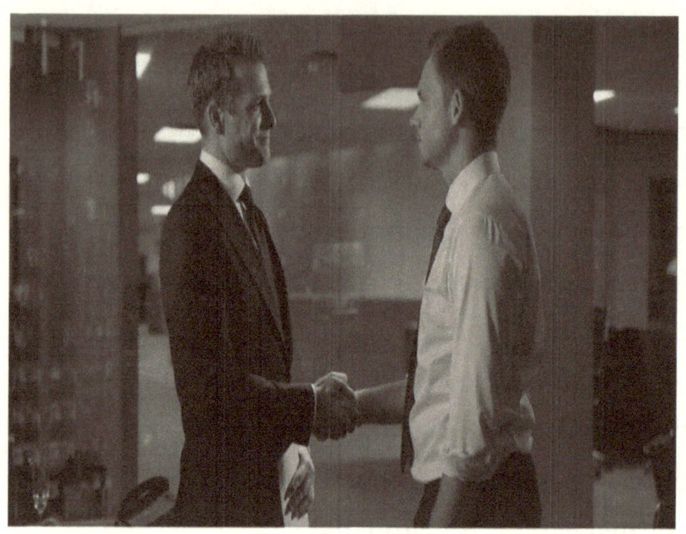

8- Nod and Smile Expectantly

Nodding is a very powerful body language tool. Whenever you're nervous, scared, or doubtful, simply nod your head and tell yourself "It's going to be ok. I've got this." This is perfect. This is a fool proof technique to seek escape from an awkward or tough situation or meeting.

9- Cross Arms or Legs

You must have probably heard that you shouldn't cross your arms as it might make you seem defensive or guarded. This goes for your legs too. Keep your arms and legs open. Cross arms or legs indirectly depict negation in a way, even if you genuinely do not mean it.

10- Don't touch your face often

Touching your face might make you seem nervous and can be distracting for the listeners or the people in the conversation. It also depicts to the second person or the audience that you are not comfortable in your skin or rather you are not comfortable the way you have groomed yourself. This leads to people observing the minute flaws which would have been not visible if not fidgeted with or unintentionally brought to notice by you.

11- Hairstyle

The hairstyle of many hotshot soccer players makes them look good on the playing field.

However, the same hairstyle might suit your lifestyle.

Find a haircut that works well with your facial bone structure, stick to it, and soon it will be a part of your personality.

The following are some recommended hair looks for men. You can choose the one most suitable to your tastes. Don't forget to take into consideration your age, work area, position, social status, and occasion.

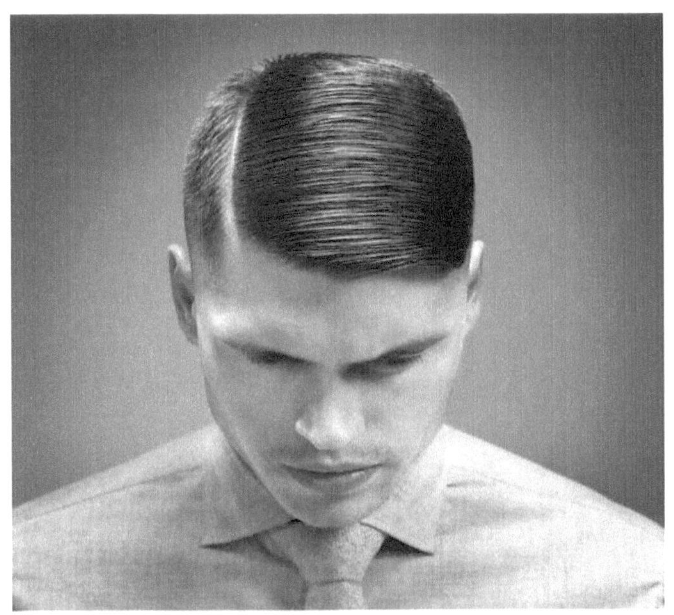

#1 Combed and Dapper Look

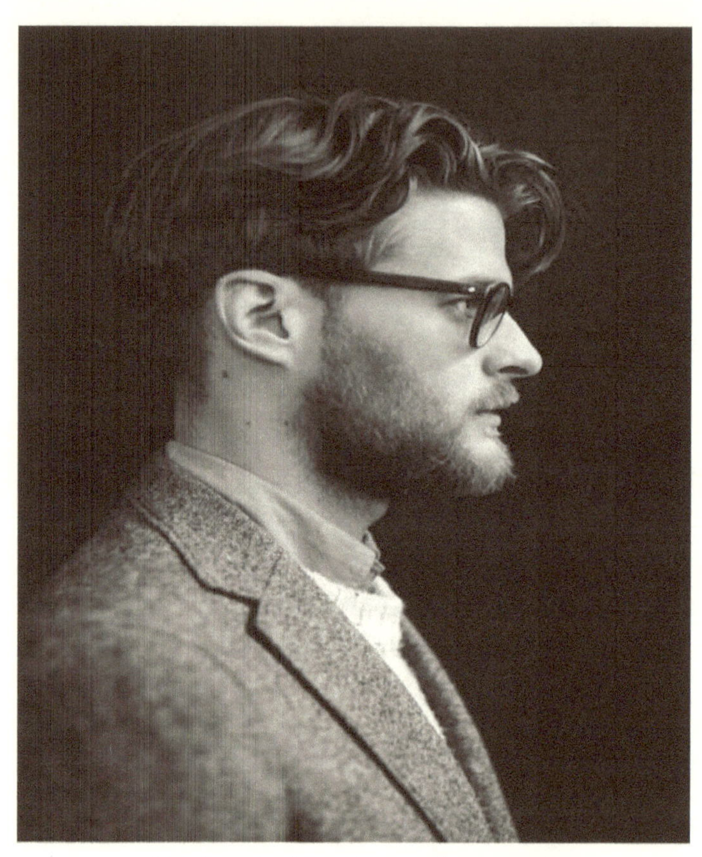

#2 Tousled and Bearded Look

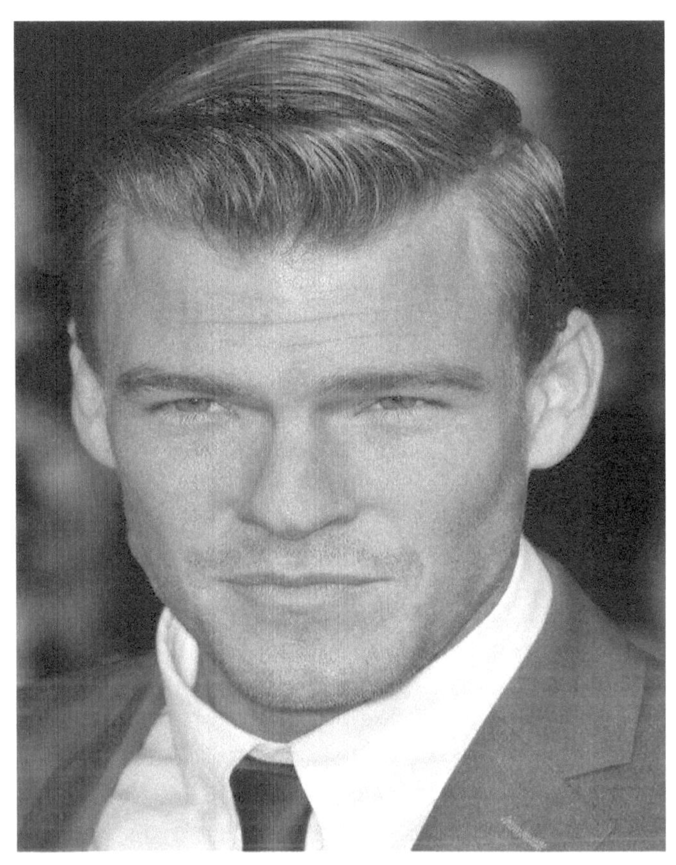

#3 Pulled Back Look

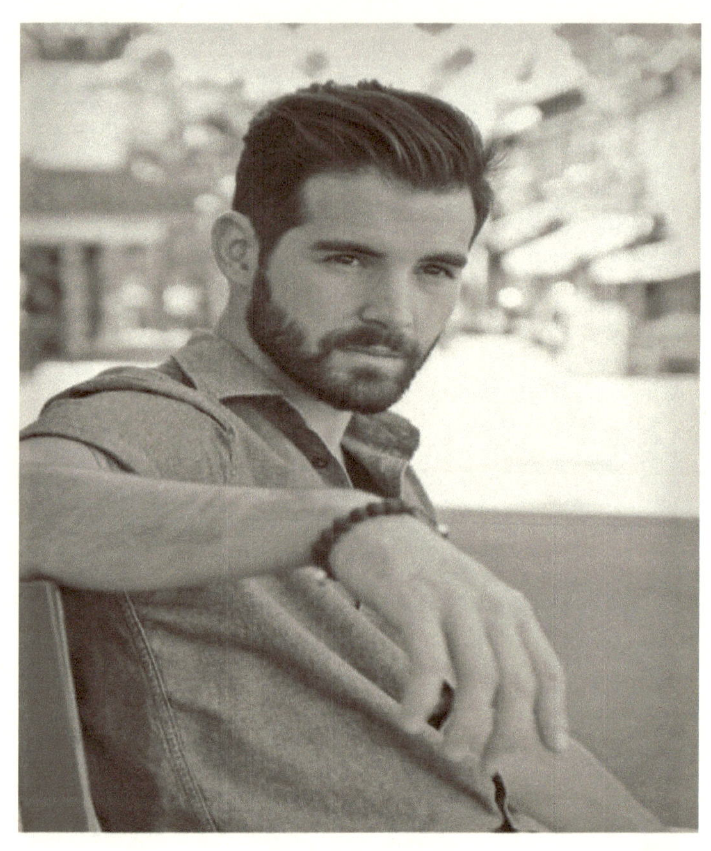

#4 Seductive Italian Style

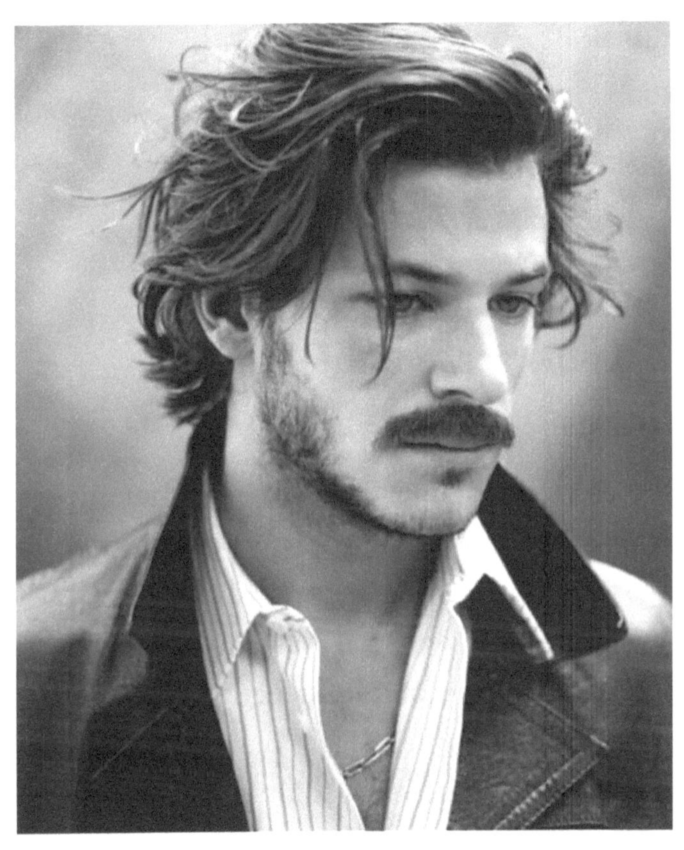

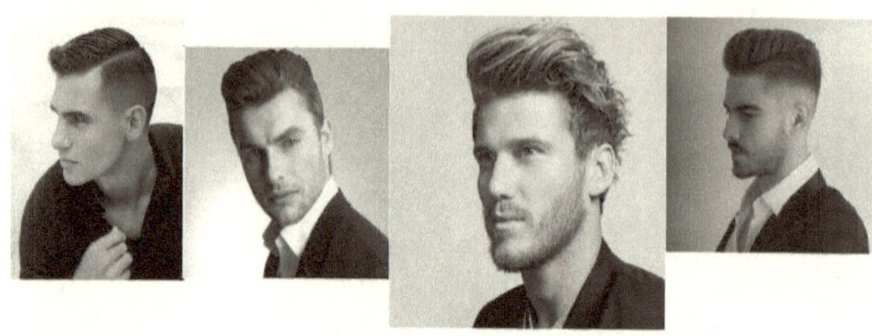

12- Look presentable in good clothes

Clothes don't define who you are, but give a glimpse into your style and purpose. You don't have to always dress in expensive clothes. With a few simple basics you can make it your tagline to successfully attract and influence people.

It is not a costly affair. Here are some easy tips and tricks for men looking to make an impression.

Tip#1

Incorporate basic colours. The choice of colors does matter a lot and also saves you a lot of money. For example, White, Black and Royal blue are universally accepted, easily available in any fabric and favorite among every gender and area of work.

It is an unwritten rule that every man must own a white and a black shirt as it goes with all types of pants, shoes and every occasion.

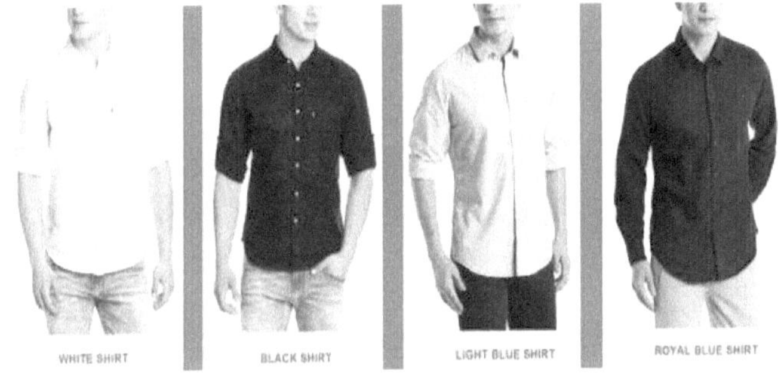

Tip#2

The T-shirt is made for a toned and muscular body.

Tight body and toned muscle is a symbol of good health. It also adds a lot to your choice of clothing. T-shirts look good on people who have a good body and toned muscles. However, very few people fall in the ideal toned category.

But it is not impossible to work for it. So, if you are skinny or have a belly, avoid wearing tight T-shirts. Either way, t-shirts will expose that. But, who wants to wear a formal shirt? This is where short sleeves-shirts come in the picture.

TIP#3

Turn your shirt into a short-sleeved shirt by simply rolling up your sleeves

Tucked in shirts look very formal. Instead, wear your shirts over your trousers.

If the length is not right, go to your tailor and get it cut lengthwise, so that it reaches a little below your waist.

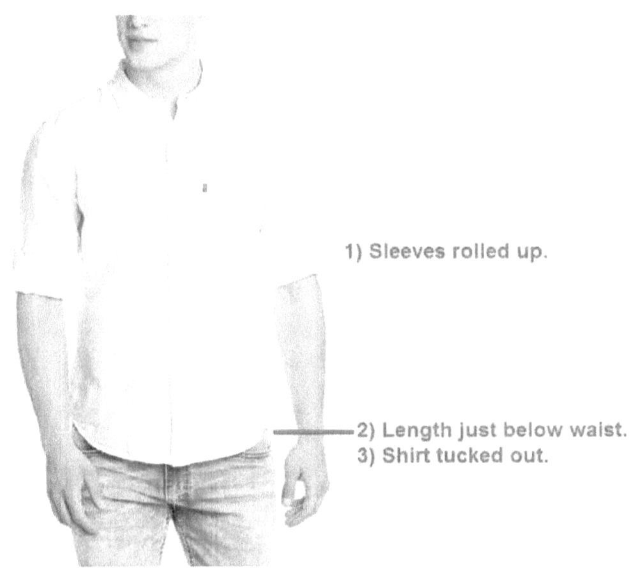

If you want to look a bit formal, just tuck them in, although because of the short length, you might need to adjust the shirt from time to time.

TIP#4

Learn to correctly roll up your sleeves.

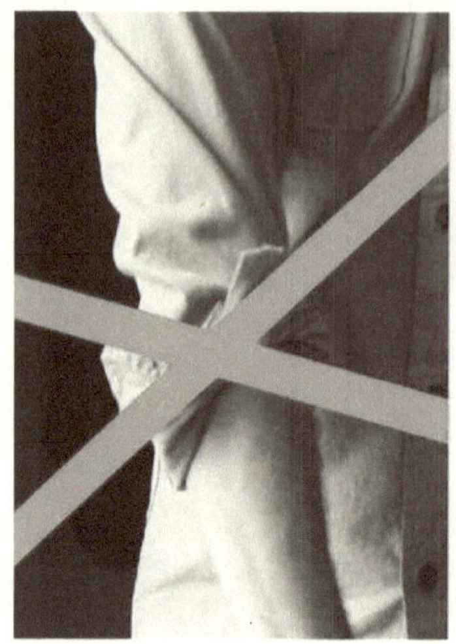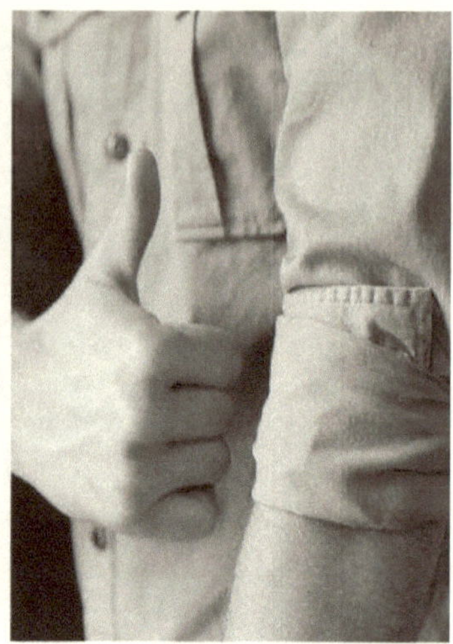

TIP#5

Grow a beard.

Not exactly a dressing hack, but it will alter your appearance. Beards accentuate your jawline and make it look sharper.

Think of how women use eyeliner to draw their eyes with "sharper" lines, your beard is your natural makeup and you can define your jaw to make it look the way you want.

Your best bet is to give your face an angular jawline. This can be tricky to get it right at home. So, visit a good salon for the first few times.

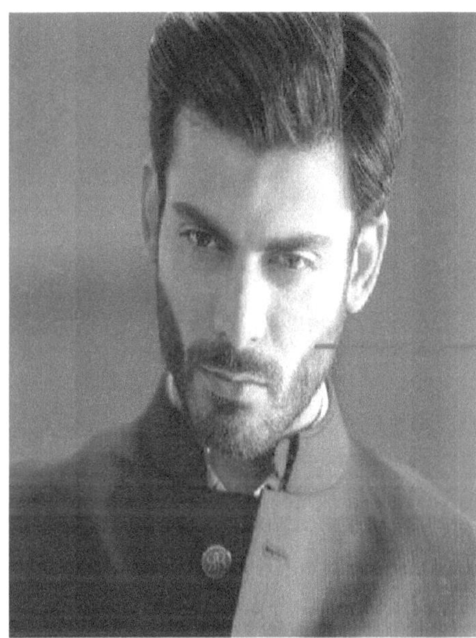

Tip #6

Wear accessories. It helps you to stand out from a crowd. These small details of the outfit perform an important role.

Whether it's a fancy watch, small bracelet or a ring, having accessories accentuates your style. Women love a man who knows how to accessorize!

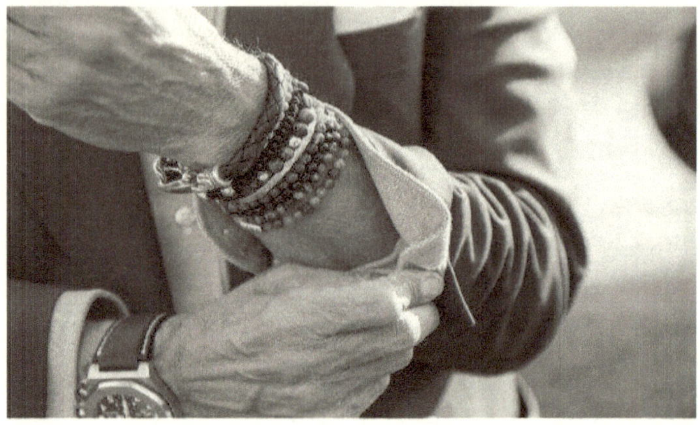

Tip #7

Slim fit T-Shirt and pants are a good combination. This is a no-brainer. You can literally wear any solid colour tee with well-fitted jeans and sneakers, boots or loafers to complete your look.

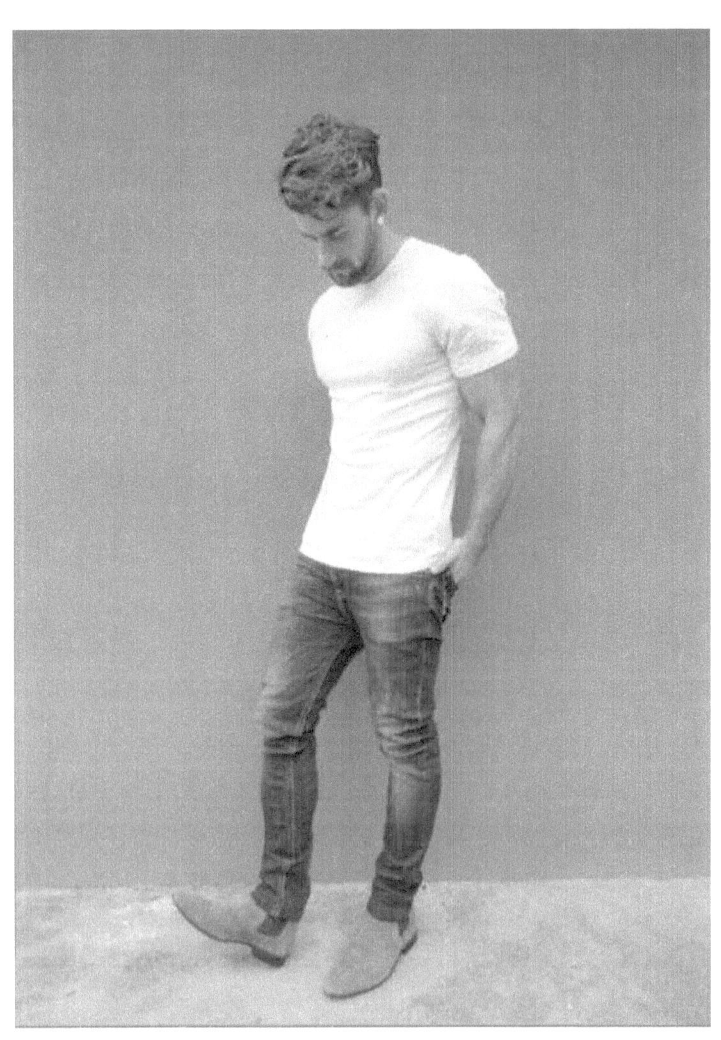

14- Keep a good attitude

Keep a positive, approachable and relaxed attitude. How you feel will come through in your body language and can make a major difference. A Warm, confident, relaxed and Supportive attitude generates healthy and warm energy vibes.

15- Take Bath with Mineral Salt

It will make your skin glow more and make you attractive. Lounging in a mineral salt bath isn't just a stress-relieving activity. It purges your body of toxins and can lead to healthier skin.

Besides this, it is a part of basic hygiene. A cleaner and healthy skin is more of a priority than clear and glowing skin.

16- Present Yourself as High Status

In 1969, University of North Carolina Sociologist Glen Elder found that looks and wealth tend to find one another — namely, good-looking women tended to settle down with less attractive but wealthier men.

Taking note from this, you should present yourself as a cultured and well-mannered individual.

Have you heard the popular saying "Fake it, till you make it". Take inspiration from this famous saying and present yourself in a manner that you aspire to be. It will definitely help you to attract people, but also influence them in the right way.

17-Wear a good cologne

It is true that fragrances have a lot to do with how you will be remembered. Make it a point to always sport a good perfume or strong cologne that will influence the people around you in a positive way.

Wearing a good cologne is synonymous with dressing well. Spraying a good perfume is the final touch to your outfit. A pleasant fragrance sets a welcoming approach and you can influence people much better. Invest in a good cologne and a deodorant so that you can keep reapplying and smelling good on the go!

18- Grooming etiquettes for men

Keep your nails short and clean (long or dirty nails mean your fingers won't get to do any exploring, *wink wink*).

1. Same goes for toenails, minus the "exploring" reason. This is just because long toenails are off-putting and makes it look like you don't take care of yourself.
2. Do not, I repeat, DO NOT shave your chest hair if you are a man. That makes intimate moments uncomfortable and prickly. Do keep the package region neatly trimmed though. Please do not shave, just manage.
3. Brush and floss teeth in the morning and before bed.
4. To sum up 3, 4 &6: Stubble anywhere but the face is a huge turn-off. Huge.
5. Stubble on the face, however, is usually sexy as hell.

6. Don't go overboard with the hair products. Use in moderation so that you can have women running their fingers through them.

7. Speaking of hair, if it's going gray, leave it as it is. Again, this is sexy. A man who dyes his hair in an attempt to hold onto his youth just screams pathetic. Women also fancy men who can rock the salt and pepper look.

19- Walk with Confidence

A man or woman of substance always beholds a style of walking that emits power and dynamicity in their character.

Remember, you don't walk in a room filled with individuals with your educational degree hanging around your neck, So, make it a point that you walk in with confidence and make yourself approachable and impressive. If you got their heads turning, then you are already breezing through the game!

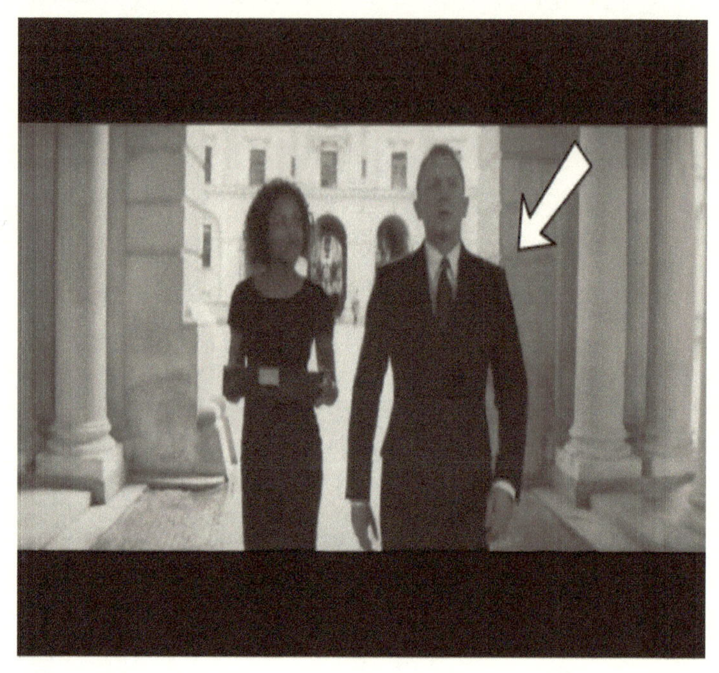

***

COMMUNICATION

1- Eyes-feet reflex

When you see someone interesting, walk towards that individual with a little smile. Right away, 98% of the time, you lose the opportunity or you creep the other individual out just by waiting.

It is also important to learn a little about reading body language. If the individual you are approaching sees you do that and happens to turn their head away or engage in a conversation out of a sudden, it is , my friends , an alarming signal to halt and look for another area of interest!

We are here to be attractive and impressive and not unpleasant and creepy.

2- Get People talking about what they Love

Get People to share what they love and they will associate you with that amazing thing. Talking constantly about yourself will give out an impression as if you are bragging about yourself. Give space to people to talk and express his/her views. This not only keeps them engaged but also increases your knowledge and sometimes happens to alter your outlook or perspective towards something. This is a fundamental of a healthy and fruitful conversation.

3- Art of Synchronization

We like people with similar interests. Try to find out similarities it may be anything like TV Series, Game, Book or anything. Try to make communication on it. It creates a huge impact for attraction. Many attractive people incorporate this in their lives.

4- 3V's Of Communication

1. Visual- Try to make the same body language.
2. Vocal- Synchronising your Voice, Tone, and Pitch with people around you will work wonders. So try to match the rhythm. Maintaining emotional level in a conversation is very essential. If the person is emotional then we also need to talk in a slow voice and maintain that pitch level too.
3. Verbal- Show interest in their story and talks.

Try to use great vocabulary that makes a great impact on people.

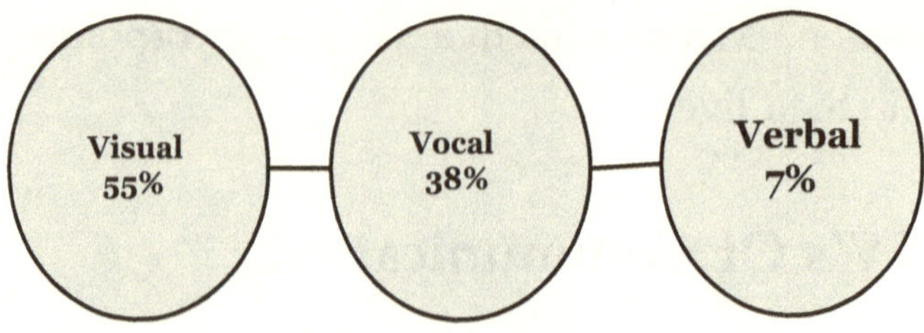

Harmony of 3V's makes us active and responsive.

5- Ask Deep Questions?

Always ask deep questions like what do you like usually? Always ask 'Wh' questions like 'who', 'what', 'when', 'where' and 'why'. That shows the person that you are on the same page and in sync with their thoughts and actions.

6- Dare to Disagree

Show them that you have funny, smart and semi-original thoughts of your own. Women tend to find men to be superficial when they agree with them on everything just to please them.

So, if you're looking to influence people, it's not a bad thing to have contrasting thoughts and opinions.

Don't be like the sheep in a herd. Dare to disagree and have unconventional ideas. Take pride in voicing them. A confident person is a great influencer who can attract the attention of anyone.

On the other hand, It is always great to stay on real opinion. Becoming attractive and impressive, in no world means to lose yourself and your thoughts.

8- If you don't have anything nice to say

If you really do not want to speak your opinion, don't say anything at all.

The words you choose to describe someone are the words that you'll be remembered for. So, if you don't have anything nice to say, it's better to stay silent.

9- Slower movements

Talk slower and deeper than normal. And like Cajun says in Beyond Words, move like you are under water.

Look at any archetypical alpha male character from a movie and the first thing that you'll notice is that they seem to do everything extra slow. Take any Clint Eastwood character for instance. He hardly says more than a few dozen words in a movie but he still looks like the coolest guy ever. In fact, researchers have found that men who have slower movements and speech are often perceived as more at ease and confident, and thus, more attractive.

When you talk slowly, you are giving more attention to the words you are saying. This makes the listener more aware of your thoughts and they find you reliable as opposed to a person who speaks hurriedly.

"In Effective Communication listening is a fine art"

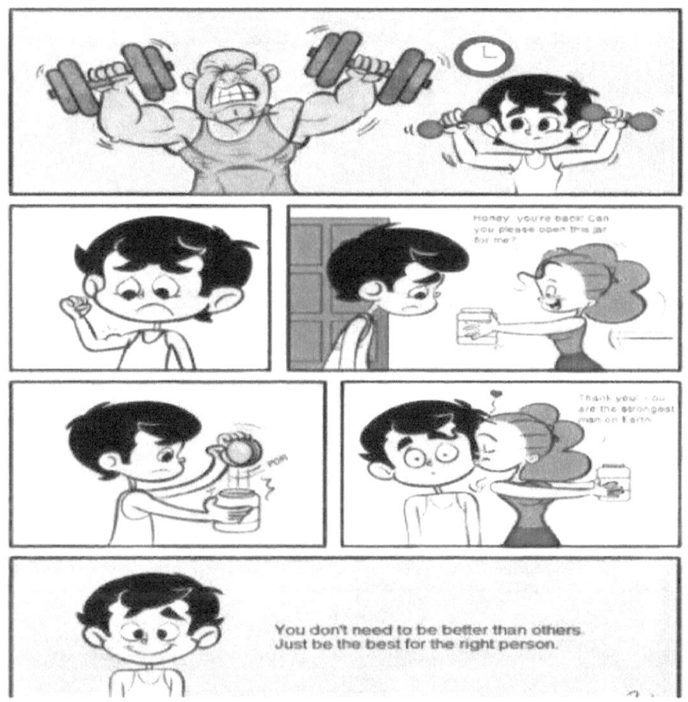

I know this might be a lot to take in. But for a while this is all that I found necessary and important for everyone like you and me. Thanks for reading these interesting facts!

Let us know in the comments below what other interesting facts you know about Human psychology.

____

____

____

____

____

____

____

____

____

____

____

____

____

____

____

____

____